Meals that help you Lose Belly Fat Fast

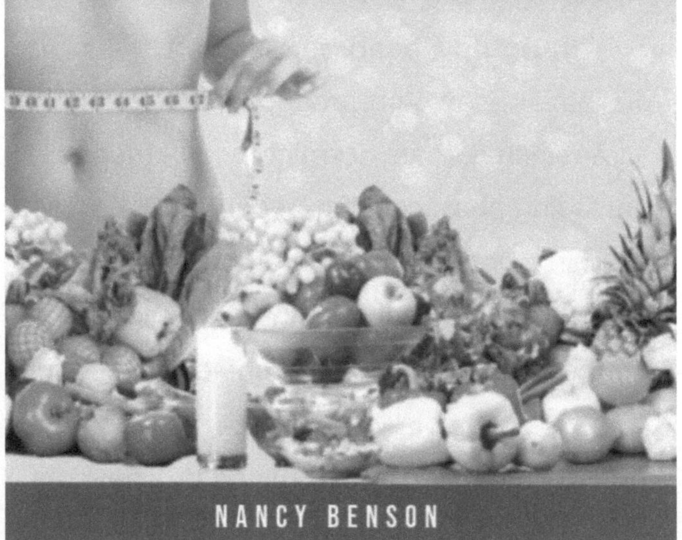

I0790748

COPYRIGHT

Nancy Benson © 2020

INTRODUCTION

If you are serious about losing belly fat, then it is important you know that diet is the most essential part of the fat loss process. With the right diet plan, which includes you eating the right foods in the right proportion, you will strip off body fat layer after layer, and say bye-bye to belly fat forever. However, if you are not following a proper diet plan, and you are eating the wrong kind of food, you will only be hindering your fat loss goal more and more.

With the wrong diet plan you will have to be acquainted with increasing your belt size notch after notch, because your belly fat will not be going away anytime soon.

In order to make sure that you are not making any mistakes with your choice of food, I want to expose you to the best foods that you should eat on a regular basis so that you can lose that belly fat in no time.

Not only do these meals aid you in losing fat quick, they also help you build lean muscle mass as well. Most of these foods are my personal favorites, so I absolutely consider these among the best diet foods for burning belly fat for both men and women.

You can as well include these foods in your personal meal plan. Have fun!

EGGS

The food I want to begin with is egg. Eggs are great to add into your diet plan because they are high in healthy fats, and protein, and they can make you feel full for a very small amount of total calories.

Eggs are also one of the most bioavailable sources of protein that is present today, which means that your body will effectively digest, absorb, and assimilate the protein present in eggs.

Having a protein source that is solid like eggs in your meals will help you in the prevention of muscle loss while you at the same time consuming less calories to create enough of a deficit to burn fat.

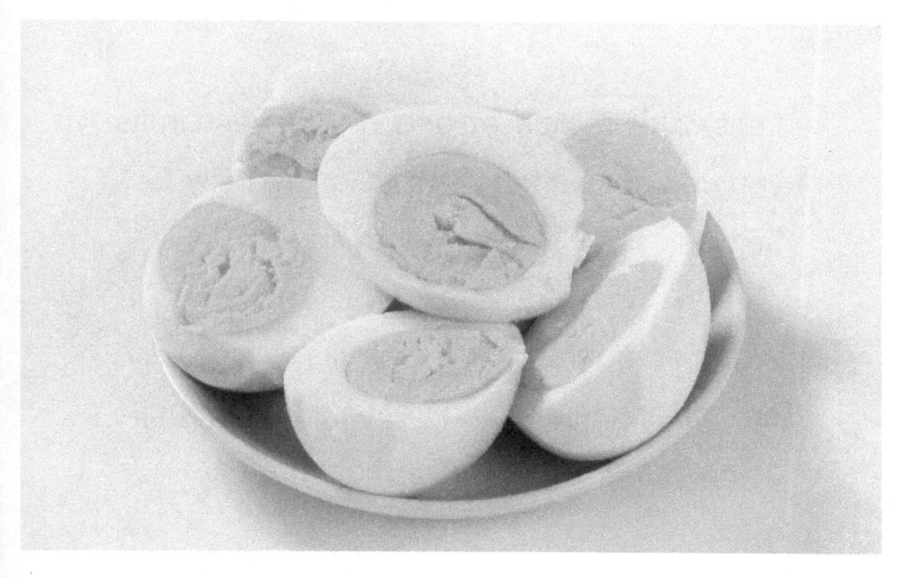

BERRIES

Let's take a look at one of the best fruits you can eat with the aim of losing belly fat - berries.

When compared to other fruits, berries are full of vitamins and antioxidants, while being extremely low in carbohydrates.

These antioxidants can help to boost blood flow which increases the delivery of oxygen to the muscles and cells generally. Overall, this can help improve your workouts, while helping with the loss of fat.

The best berries to eat are the ones which have low carb and they are; blackberries, blueberries, and raspberries.

Blueberries have a slightly higher amount of carbs contained in them, so in order to keep the intake of calories low, you should stick with blackberries and raspberries.

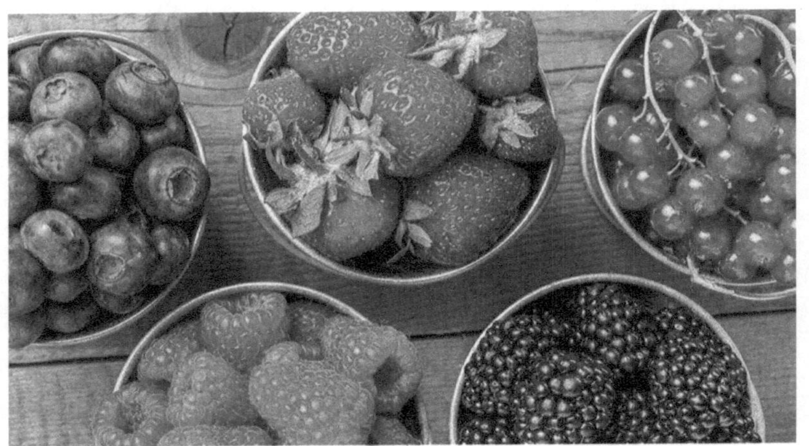

AVOCADO

Unlike other fruits which contain so much carbohydrate, Avocados are loaded with healthy monounsaturated fats, specifically oleic acid. They also contain enough fiber which will make you feel full for a longer period.

One other fascinating thing about avocados that was found during a research from The Ohio State University in Columbus is that avocados aid in the absorption of 15x more carotenoids from vegetables and fruits.

Avocados will not only help you burn fat, but you will also be making your immune system more powerful as you will be absorbing more cancer fighting carotenoids than you did before.

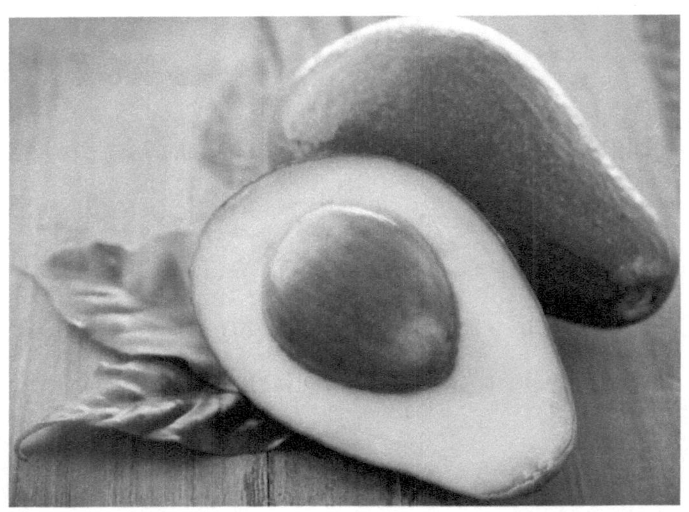

APPLE CIDER VINEGAR

Apple cider vinegar isn't actually a food, but instead it is a drink which has been discovered to be very efficient in helping to reduce belly fat.

Studies have shown that apple cider vinegar helps people lose weight along with a reduction in their waist circumference. These are not the regular animal studies that you often see which do not actually guarantee the same results for humans, contrary these are human studies.

One of these studies spanned upto 12 weeks and it showed that obese persons had the ability to lose weight anywhere from 2.7 to 3.8 pounds just by taking 1 to 2 tablespoons of apple cider vinegar daily.

Apple cider vinegar has also been discovered to improve blood sugar spikes after meals, and it can aid in enhancing fullness after a meal.

To be precise, on study showed that adding apple cider vinegar to a meal with high carb content could make one eat 200 to 280 less calories in a day.

Bear in mind, you want to ensure that you do not drink it straight up, instead you dilute only 1 to 2 teaspoons of apple cider vinegar in water.

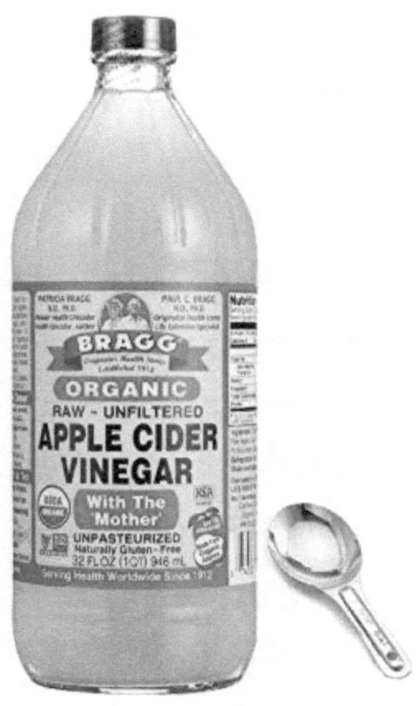

PATRICIA BRAGG
N.D., Ph.D.
Noted Health Crusader
Health Educator, Author
PAUL C. BRAGG
N.D., Ph.D.
Originator Health Food
Life Extension Specialist
BRAGG
Organic Health Stores
Established 1912
ORGANIC
RAW - UNFILTERED
APPLE CIDER
VINEGAR
With The
Mother
UNPASTEURIZED
Naturally Gluten-Free
32 FL OZ (1QT) 946 mL
Serving Health Worldwide Since 1912

TUNA

Tuna is another high protein food that aids in the reduction of fat. It is a lean fish which is basically made up of protein - this makes tuna a massive route to increase the consumption of protein without having to increase the intake of calories.

One vital thing to remember is that when buying canned tuna, you want to ensure that you do not buy the tuna in oil but the one in water, the reason is because if you get tuna in oil then all the extra calories that you do not consume from the low fat fish [tuna] will be override by the oil.

Fishes generally are a great option for trying to burn fat.

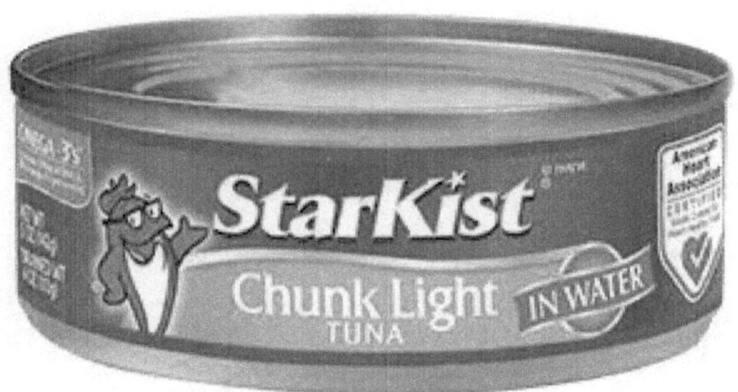
StarKist
Chunk Light
TUNA
IN WATER
OMEGA-3's

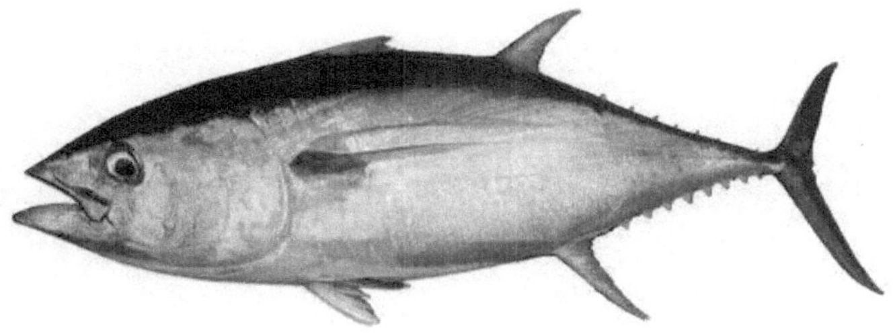

SALMON

Salmon is filled with high quality protein - healthy omega 3 fatty acids which helps lower inflammation, and it also contains several other important nutrients. It also gives a full feeling and contains iodine, which is an essential nutrient for proper thyroid function to make sure that your metabolism is functioning at its best form.

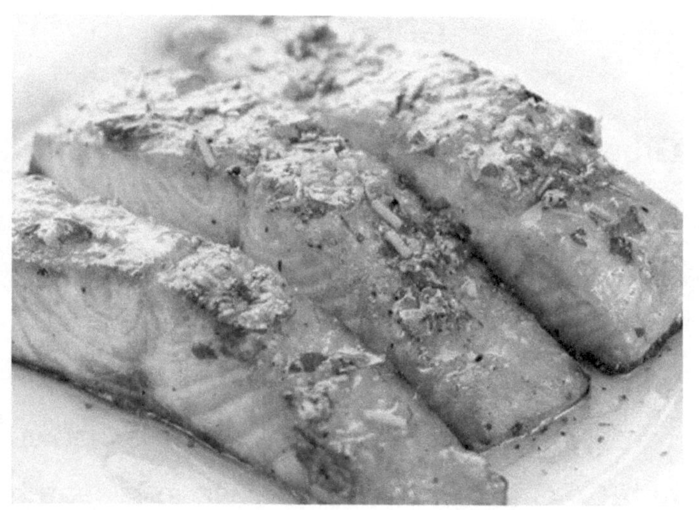

GREEN TEA

Green tea is a drink which can help speed up your fat burning process, please do not get me wrong, sitting at a spot and drinking green tea alone all day is not going to make you lose belly fat. However, green tea contains a compound in it which is known as ECGC that has been shown in research to aid increase in fat loss.

Three cups of green tea daily or the addition of ECGC to a supplement can boost your fat loss, especially when combined with a proper diet plan and exercise program.

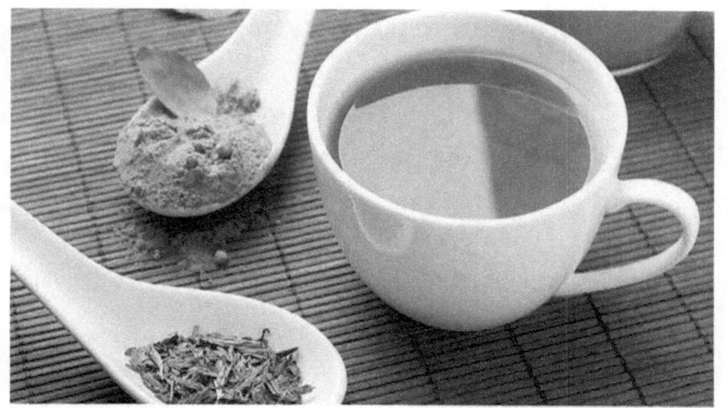

LEAFY GREEN VEGETABLES

In order to have a healthy diet plan, one food that you should be adding to your diet which I should have actually began with are leafy green vegetables. They include swiss chards, collard greens, kale and spinach, and a bit more.

Green vegetables generally are a good method of decreasing hunger and increasing fullness, they are also not densed with so much caloric content. The feeling of fullness comes from the volume of leafy green vegetables you consume as well as the fiber present inside the leafy green vegetables.

Added to the feeling of fullness for a very little caloric cost, green leafy vegetables are loaded with beta-carotene, and plenty of minerals and vitamins.

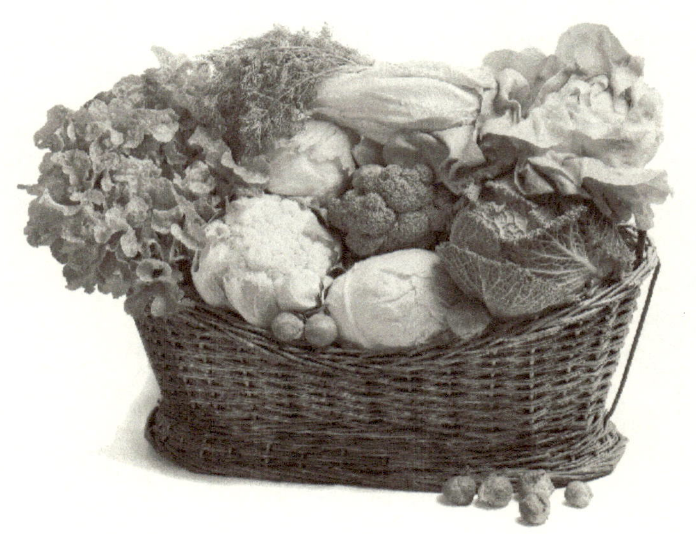

CHICKEN BREAST

Chicken breast just like tuna is a very lean source of protein that makes you feel full for a little amount of calories. Consuming plenty of protein the entire day like eggs, salmon, chicken breast, and tunas have been shown in research to reduce cravings upto 60%.

Reducing your cravings is one of the best methods of preventing late night binge eating, which is a major part of the fight for a smaller waistline.

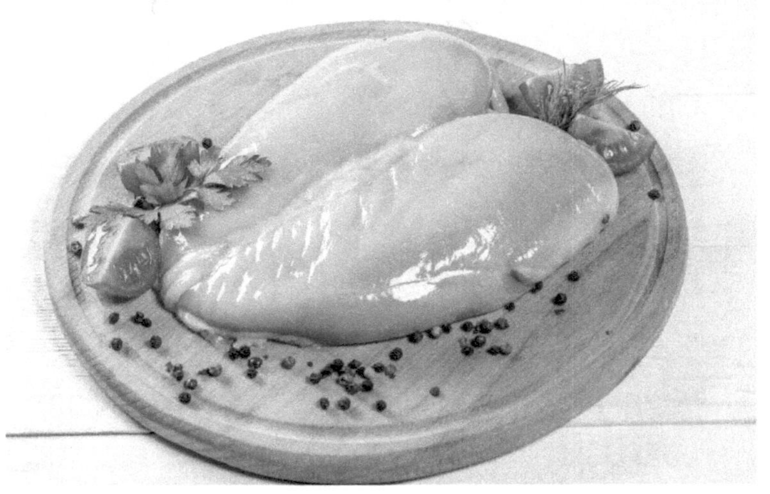

SWEET POTATOES

Sweet potatoes have a fairly low caloric content, and they are slow digesting as well, so you will be full for a longer amount of time.

One other reason why sweet potatoes are great at keeping you full is because they contain a large quantity of dietary fiber which occupies a lot of room in your stomach and as a result stops you from overeating.

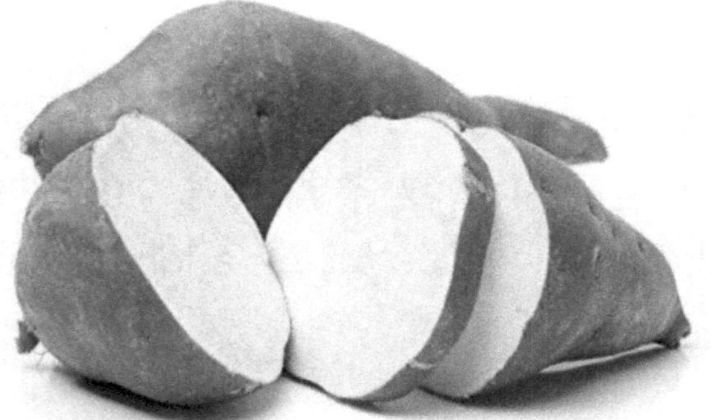

OATMEAL

Oatmeal is also a slow digesting carb which is full of fiber that will leave you feeling full for a decent amount of time.

Also, oatmeal helps in improving digestion, which can be very essential if you are on a diet which is high in protein.

Although oats are great, you have to be cautious because not every oat is manufactured using the same method. Flavored instant oats contain plenty of added sugar, and obviously that will not in any way help you lose so much fat. Instead of eating flavored instant oats, try getting plain oatmeal and flavor it by yourself with something like cinnamon.

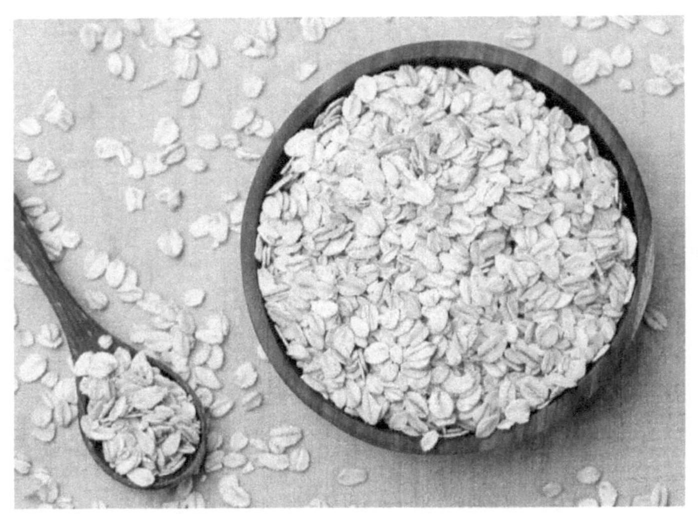

BEANS

Beans are another great carbohydrate source for losing belly fat. Beans are among the highest protein plant based foods known, so quite a lot of people think that it is in the category of protein source.

Moreover, beans with the highest protein content like black beans has much more carbohydrates than protein, so they are still basically categorized under carbohydrate source.

Irrespective of what your prior knowledge, beans are a great carbohydrate source because they contain so much fiber and protein.

There are now much more bean based products available in the market that you can add to your diet plan also. Things like black burger bean, bean potato chips, as well as black bean pasta are all worth taking a look at if you intend making your diet more versatile and enjoyable.

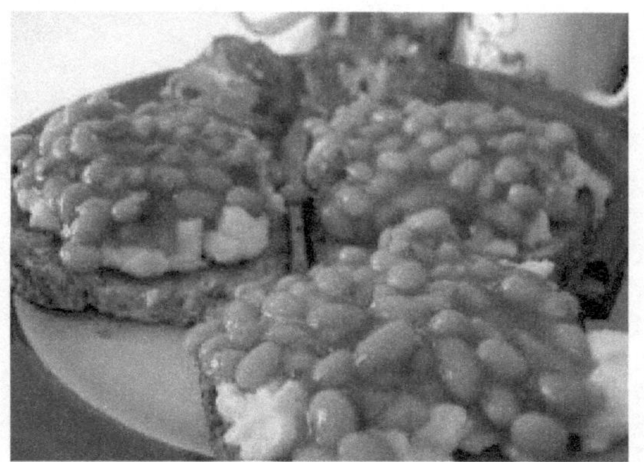

BROWN RICE

Another carb that I want to mention is actually one of my favorite carbs to eat because it helps in building muscles as well as enhancing fat burn. Like oatmeals and sweet potatoes, brown rice contains a lot of fiber, it is slow digesting, and also contains so much resistant starch - which helps in boosting metabolism and fat burn.

Studies have shown that a half cup serving of brown rice is equivalent to 1.7 grams of resistant starch.

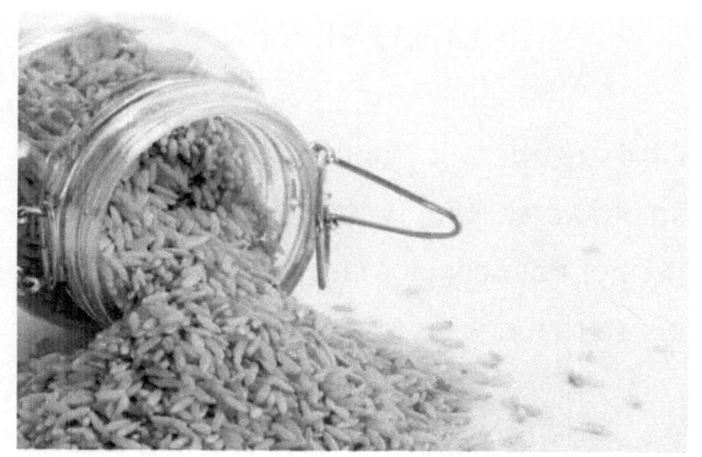

CHILLI PEPPER

Chili pepper is one food you should incorporate into your diet. Eating chili pepper not only increases your metabolism, it also reduces your appetite.

Studies have shown that for people who do not eat chilli pepper on a regular basis, eating only 1 gram of red chilli pepper reduced appetite and increased fat burning.

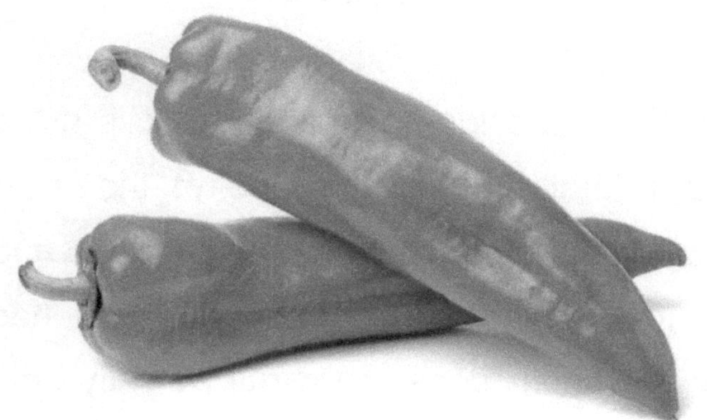

GRAPEFRUIT

Let us take a look at grapefruit. It is not a secret that grapefruit is one of the most recommended fruits by many dieticians and fat loss diet plans, but the question has always been "does grapefruit actually help in weight loss, or is it just one of the many fat dieting schemes".

A twelve-week long research was carried out on 90 people who were overweight [obese], during the research peroid, they ate ½ a grapefruit before their meals, and from tests carried out, it actually resulted in loss of about 3 to 5 pounds, and there was also in improvement in insulin sensitivity.

Why grapefruit should be an essential part of your diet plan if you intend reducing belly fat is that less insulin resistance makes it easier to burn fat faster, and eating grapefruit improves insulin sensitivity in the body.

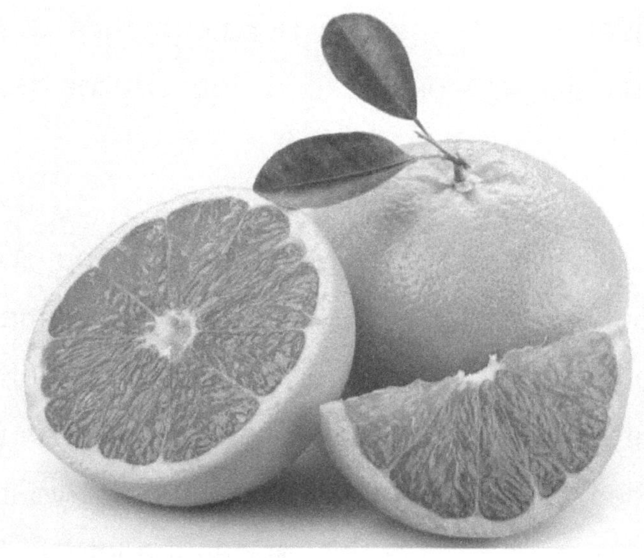

SOUP

Soup is another good food to take when you want to reduce belly fat faster. Taking soup prior to meals will help reduce the total quantity of the food you eat for the day.

Actually, it is very necessary that you do not just eat any random soup, as some soups have an extremely high carbohydrate, and high caloric content, and when you add things like croutons to your soup, your meal no longer has the intent of helping you lose belly fat.

It is advisable that you stick to low calorie soups like mushroom clear soup, vegetable soup, or chicken soup.

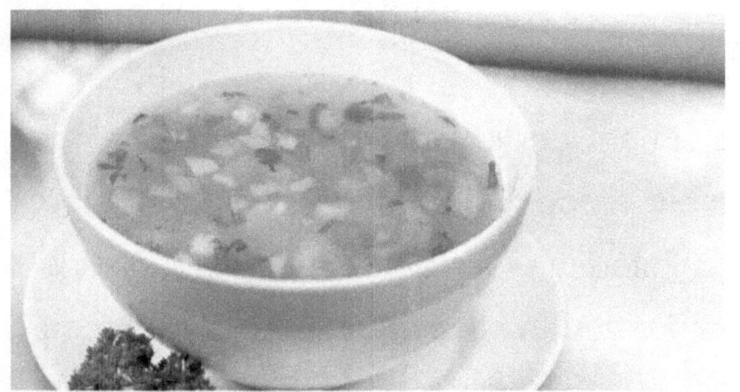

PROTEIN POWDER

Protein powder is another food which is not entirely food in reality, but can be substituted in place of a meal. Although it is ideal for you to always try to have real food over supplements, protein powder can actually help you out when you are in a fix and you do not have time to prepare an actual meal.

Protein powder is a great supplement to have after a workout if you are in need of a fast digesting protein source that will get your muscles and blood stream to begin the repairing process.

One other thing you can do with protein powder is to make a protein shake and take it before going out at a restaurant to eat with your family or friends. Consuming the protein shake will greatly reduce your hunger which will in turn reduce the quantity of food you end up eating at the restaurant.

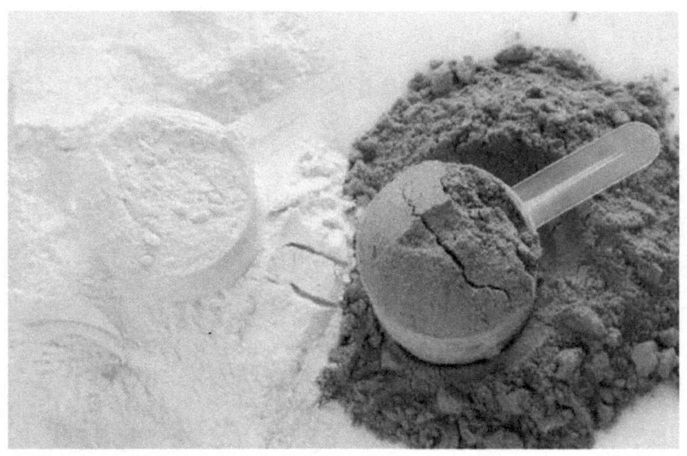

COFFEE

Enjoying the appetite suppressing effects of coffee is a great way to further reduce your hunger. Coffee is not actually a food but it is more of an empty calorie beverage which reduces you craving for food.

Black coffee is the best, and even though you add a little bit of unsweetened almond milk, or cream, you will still experience its benefits without any downside.

People who are doing an intermittent fasting use coffee as a staple because it is so effective at suppressing appetite. Many people do not know that coffee also contains several antioxidants.

One of the antioxidants present in coffee is chlorogenic acid or CGA, and it can increase the use of fat for energy in your body. Studies have shown that CGA can slow down the release of glucose and reduce insulin resistance which lowers weight gain after eating.

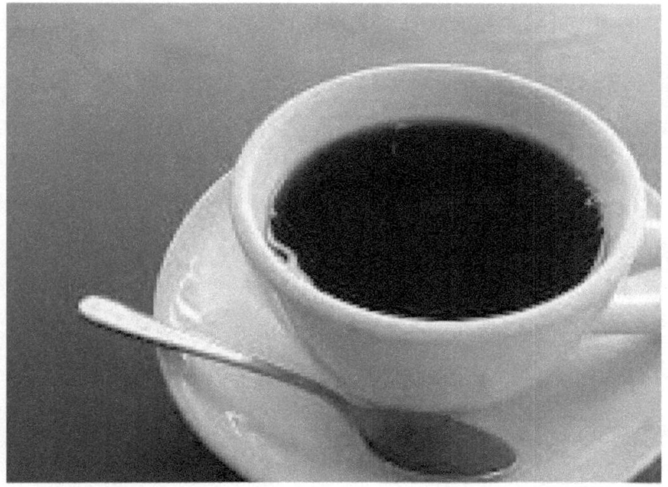

ASPARAGUS

Asparagus is the next food present on our list. Asparagus is not just a rich green vegetable which helps fill your stomach up and satisfy hunger, but studies in the past has also shown that asparagus can reduce bloating, especially around the mid region of the body.

Asparagus is one of the vegetables that are very low in carbohydrates as it only has about half a gram of carbohydrates per spear.

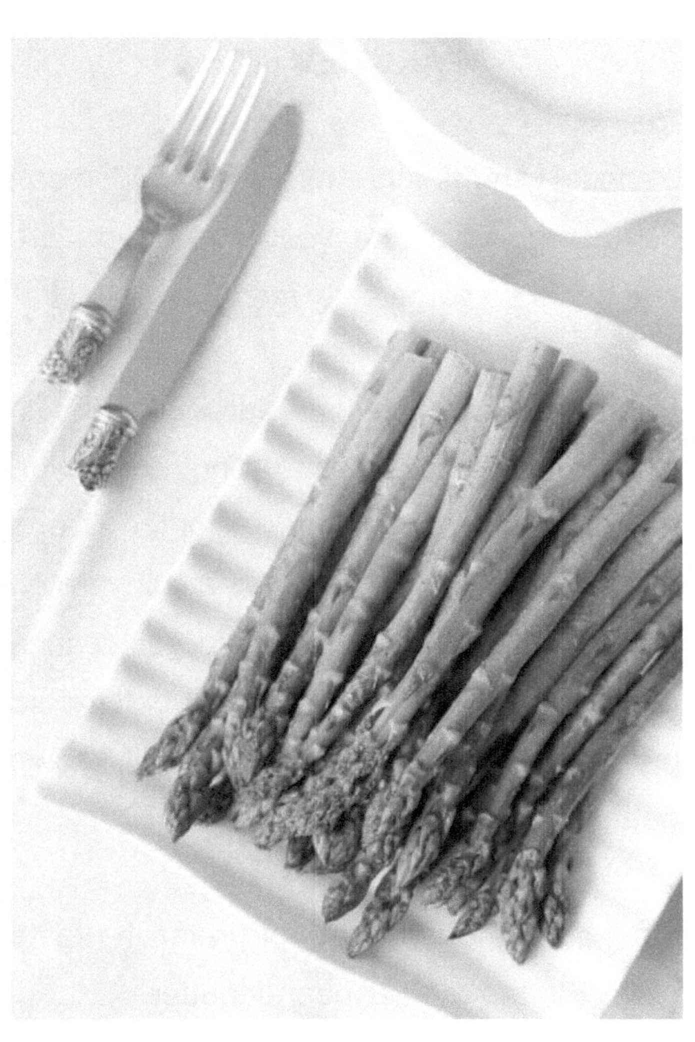

PEANUT BUTTER

Peanut butter is more of a snack which can be incorporated into your diet if you are trying to lose some belly fat.

Peanut butter contains a large amount of protein, and it is very filling. However, regular peanut butter has so much fat and caloric content, so going for a dehydrated peanut butter like PB2 can aid you reduce the calories in half while still getting so much protein and keeping that still known peanut butter taste.

Most people often than not prefer the taste of PB2 to the regular peanut butter.

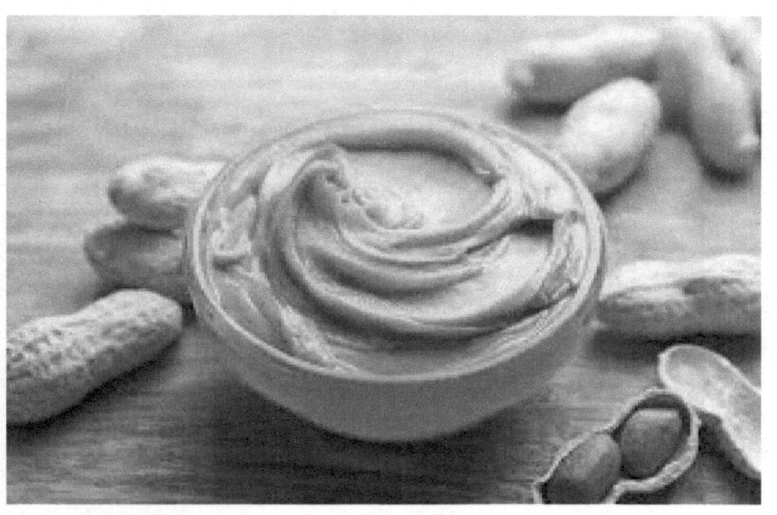

CONCLUSION

There you have it. I hope throughout the course of you reading this book, you have gotten knowledge of some of the foods which you can add to your diet to lose belly fat.

Remember, eating any or all of these foods will not necessarily equate to you losing belly fat except for the rest of your diet is on point. To lose belly fat you need to be on a diet which incorporates these foods while giving your body the needed amount of calories and increasing insulin levels.